brain boosting food for women with adhd

IMPROVE CONCENTRATION, MOTIVATION, MOOD, AND MEMORY

ESTELLE ROSE

ROSALI PUBLISHING

Copyright © 2023 by Estelle Rose - All rights reserved.

No part of this publication may be reproduced, stored or transmitted in any form or by any means, electronic, mechanical, photocopying, recording, scanning, or otherwise without written permission from the publisher. It is illegal to copy this book, post it to a website, or distribute it by any other means without permission. Estelle Rose asserts the moral right to be identified as the author of this work.

This book is copyright protected. This book is only for personal use. You cannot amend, distribute, sell, use, quote or paraphrase any part, or the content within this book, without the consent of the author or publisher.

Under no circumstances will any blame or legal responsibility be held against the publisher, or author, for any damages, reparation, or monetary loss due to the information contained within this book. Either directly or indirectly. You are responsible for your own choices, actions, and results.

Designations used by companies to distinguish their products are often claimed as trademarks. All brand names and product names used in this book and on its cover are trade names, service marks, trademarks and registered trademarks of their respective owners. The publishers and the book are not associated with any product or vendor mentioned in this book. None of the companies referenced within the book have endorsed the book.

Please note the information contained within this document is for educational and entertainment purposes only. All effort has been executed to present accurate, up to date, and reliable, complete information. No warranties of any kind are declared or implied. Readers acknowledge that the author is not engaging in the rendering of legal, financial, medical or professional advice. The content within this book has been derived from various sources. Please consult a licensed professional before attempting any techniques outlined in this book.

By reading this document, the reader agrees that under no circumstances is the author responsible for any losses, direct or indirect, which are incurred as a result of the use of the information contained within this document, including, but not limited to, — errors, omissions, or inaccuracies.

Second edition

"If you are always trying to be normal, you will never know how amazing you can be."

DR. MAYA ANGELOU

praise for estelle rose
ON "EMPOWERED WOMEN WITH ADHD"

"I have never felt so seen before and understood!"

TABITHA W.

"This book is a delightful read that merges practical advice with heartfelt wisdom. Written like a conversation with a trusted friend, its engaging illustrations and uplifting insights truly celebrate the joys of neurodiversity, guiding readers to harness ADHD as an asset."

T. SVEDMAN

"I was diagnosed as an adult in my early 30s and read the books recommended by my therapist, which were helpful but long, dry, and not specific to the challenges unique to women. I wish I had this book back then! It is full of tips, lists of strategies, and resources such as apps, all presented in an ADHD-friendly format! Visually, the book is a pure pleasure to read!"

MANDA M.

"It's always a struggle for me to read books for the simple fact I struggle with ADHD!!! Not the case with this one! This book was engaging! It helped me to learn things on a level I can understand!!! She was speaking to me, about me, and with me for sure!!!"

CARLA R.

"The thing I loved the most about this book was how personal it was. Not only does the author share relatable experiences, she also provides helpful tips for everyday life. As a mother to a daughter diagnosed with ADHD - I found this book to be incredibly helpful and empowering. It's short, but SO full of helpful information."

ALLYSON R.

"This book feels like having a highly informed conversation and a hug from a friend. It is so thoughtful in its approach and is such an easy, pleasant read. The author has personal experience with late-diagnosis ADHD and has the goal of truly helping empower other women with ADHD by sharing everything she has learned along the way."

AMANDA A.

"I have discovered I have ADHD. After becoming a mother, I have progressively become worse. I was skeptical, in denial, perhaps misunderstanding the whole diagnosis. This book helps me see it for what it is, and accept that I am running a totally different ship, an empowered one, not a helpless one."

SIMONA B.

"I cannot give this book enough praise. It was easy to read, insightful and I am grateful for the information it was able to provide me with. I cannot recommend it enough!! A must-read."

VANESSA R.

contents

Introduction	ix
1. What Not To Eat	1
2. How To Eat	5
3. Wholesome To Be Awesome	9
4. The Life-Changing Change	13
5. The Unlikely Sidekick	21
6. No Beauty Without Color	25
7. The Helpful Treat	29
8. What To Drink	31
9. How To Create Unbreakable Habits	35
10. Meal Plan	41
Conclusion	53
How To Leave A Review	55
About the Author	59
Also By Estelle Rose	61
Resources	65

introduction

Once upon a time, all the way back in 2009, a group of scientists decided to check whether a change in diet would have an impact on ADHD symptoms. So they took 27 children, all diagnosed with ADHD, and split them into two groups. How exactly? I'm not entirely sure. My guess is that it wasn't 13.5 on each side, or that wouldn't be very ethical.

Anyways, one group tried an elimination diet, and the control group kept their usual diet. After nine weeks, they asked parents and teachers if they had noticed any improvement in the children's behavior. And guess what? 73% of parents and 70% of teachers saw an improvement in the kids on the special diet, while no improvement was found in the control group. So, the scientists published their study in the *European Child & Adolescent Psychiatry* journal.

Now, we're not children, and we don't have a parent or a teacher to rate our behavior. Or do we? I don't know about you, but personally, I'm up for grabbing all the help I can. So, let me tell you a little bit about why I've been wanting to share this book with you.

While waiting for my ADHD diagnosis, I started looking into things I could do to help me in the meantime. I tried a few things, but changing my diet had the most significant impact. After only a week or two of applying the principles I'm going to share with you, I felt as if a veil had been lifted and emerged out of the fog. Don't get me wrong: I still lose my keys regularly, I still drift off in some conversations because my mind is busy elsewhere, and I still interrupt people when they talk. But I can concentrate better, and my mood and motivation have improved.

Before we get any further, I need to put a disclaimer here. I have no opinion on ADHD medication, and I respect people who choose to medicate and those who choose not to. This book shouldn't be taken as medical advice, and if you have any concerns about managing your ADHD, please speak to a psychiatrist, which I am not.

What I am is a woman with ADHD, one of those late diagnoses ones, and following this diet is one of the best things I've ever done for myself. So, I am writing this book as a peer, as a friend who wants you to experience the same life-changing improvements. Food doesn't give you ADHD. And food doesn't 'cure' ADHD. Nothing does, and in my opinion, that's probably a good thing. But if it helps me and many others manage symptoms, it can help you whether you are on medication or not.

Numerous studies show the impact of nutrition on conditions such as Alzheimer's and depression, and guess what? ADHD is no different. A systematic review and meta-analysis of studies published in the journal *Clinical Nutrition* in 2019 has shown that "a "Healthy" dietary pattern [...] has decreased the odds of ADHD up to 37%."

What you put into your body impacts your brain. This is overall a very healthy diet, and following it might also help the people you're living with simply by modeling a healthier lifestyle. They don't have to be women or have ADHD to benefit from it.

There are additional benefits, too. If weight is an issue for you as it was for me, chances are you will lose weight in the process. I have lost 40 pounds and have kept the weight off since making these changes. I have always had a very complicated relationship with food. I've only recently realized how strongly it was linked to my ADHD. In my case, I think it was both a way to self-harm and a simple way to boost my dopamine level with constant small gratifications throughout the day.

If the words "diet" and "elimination" scare you, don't be afraid: it is not about going 'on a diet'; it is about implementing some changes to what you're eating to give your brain a helping hand. Of course, how big or small these changes are will depend on what your current diet looks like and how much you want to change, so let's dive in.

Another disclaimer is that my mother tongue is French. I live in England and am trying to write in American English. So, I apologize for the possible weird idioms and turns of phrases you might find in this book.

SPECIAL GIFTS FOR YOU

GRAB THEM NOW

Follow this link:
bit.ly/brainboostingrecipes

Or scan the QR code

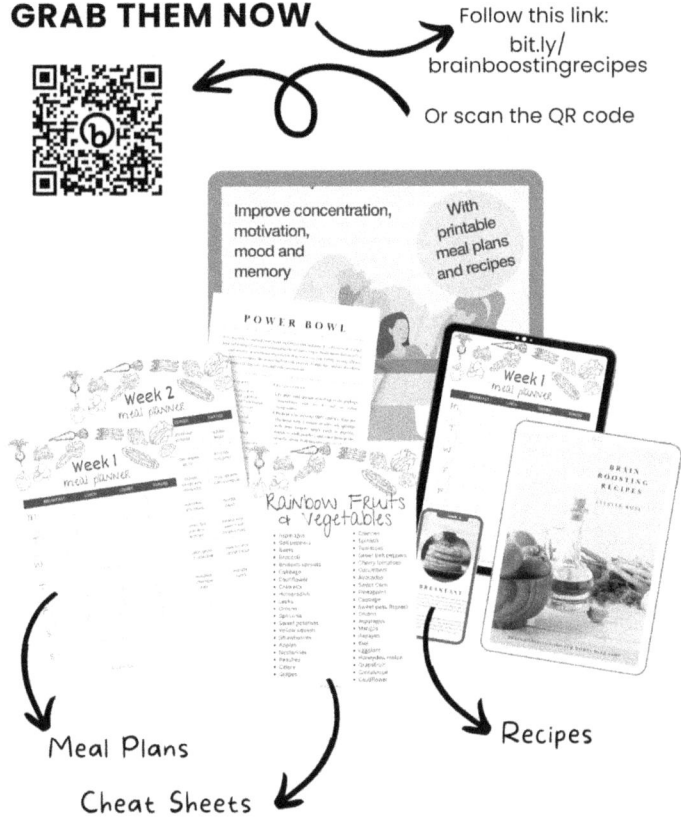

Meal Plans

Cheat Sheets

Recipes

Print or use them with any PDF Annotation App

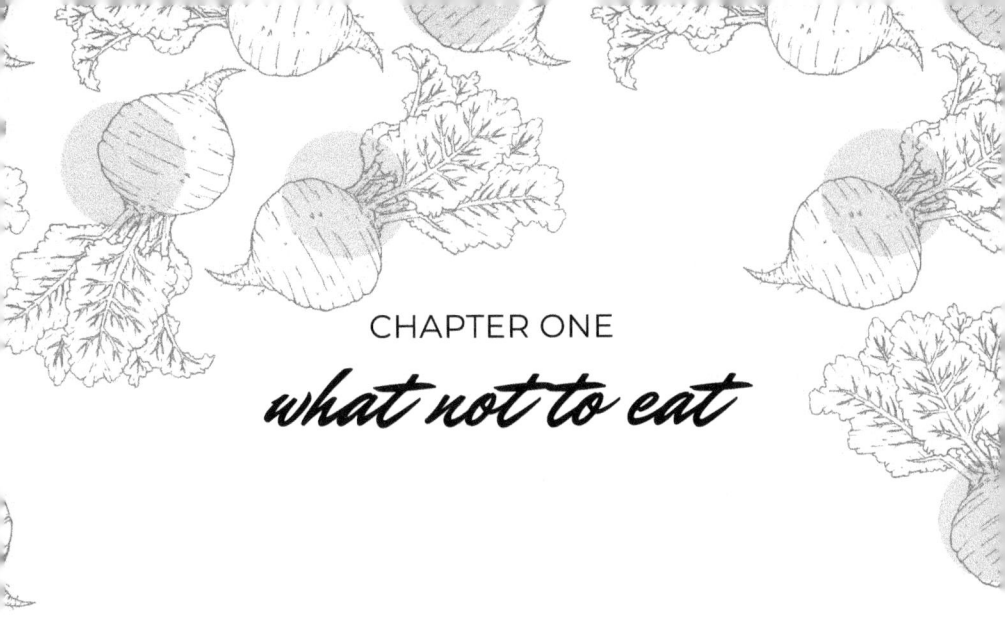

CHAPTER ONE
what not to eat

OKAY, so before I share the brain-boosting foods that will help your beautiful ADHD brain thrive, we need to discuss what might harm it. Unfortunately, some foods are making things worse, and I'm going to help you identify how many of those you are consuming at the moment.

Processed Food

Processed food is any food that you buy already prepared or that has been transformed before you buy it. So it can be as simple as frozen food or tinned food. While those are okay to use for convenience (I'm not a monster), you definitely want to stay clear of highly processed foods, which include:

- Sweet snacks
- Savory snacks
- Packaged meat: sausage, bacon, salami, ham, etc.
- Ready meals

Not only do they contain too much of all the usual unhealthy baddies (sugar, salt, unhealthy fat), but they often also contain additives that may worsen ADHD symptoms. It's a hot debate that has been going on since 1975. Still, following recent studies, the American Academy of Pediatrics agrees that children with ADHD should eliminate the following from their diets:

- Artificial colors
- Aspartame
- MSG (monosodium glutamate)
- Nitrites
- Sodium benzote

I know we're not children, but we can benefit from not eating those too.

SUGAR

Sorry, I had to drop the 'S word'. A study by Robert Prinz in the *Journal of Consulting and Clinical Psychology* concluded that the more sugar children eat, the more restless they become. And another one at Yale University showed a link between sugar and inattention. And that's on children without ADHD. So imagine what it can do to our already restless minds.

Personally, I still eat cake... sometimes. But the sugar we can all get rid of is hidden and unnecessary, and you're not even really enjoying it. I've already mentioned it in processed food. If you do buy tinned food for convenience, please check the label. Actually, you probably want to check the label of everything that is not fresh fruits or vegetables. Here are some examples of the most common foods with hidden sugars:

- Cereals
- Some oatmeal
- Flavored yogurt
- (Not so healthy) granola bars
- Dried fruits
- Sauces: ketchup, BBQ sauce, pasta sauce

You also want to be careful not to drink your sugar and avoid sugary drinks. These include sodas, energy drinks, fruit juice, and when you add sugar or syrup to your tea or coffee.

Elimination Diet

You don't have to do it, but this could be a life-changing improvement. Let me explain.

First, what is an elimination diet? It is less complicated than it may sound, and you don't need specialist help to do it. You simply need to conduct an experiment with your diet by removing one kind of food at a time and paying attention to changes in how you feel.

People with ADHD can benefit from going through this, as some studies have shown a link between food intolerance and loss of focus and hyperactivity. The most common food intolerances you might want to test are:

- Gluten
- Wheat
- Corn
- Soy
- Dairy

I tested these and realized that I am intolerant to wheat. I feel sooooo much better when I don't have it. But because it is only an intolerance, I'm okay if I have cake once in a while. What I shouldn't do is have jam on toast for breakfast, an avocado sandwich for lunch, and tomato pasta for dinner.

If you're keen to try this method, here is how to proceed:

1. Identify which food you want to test first. You might already suspect that a particular food is causing you trouble. If you don't know what to test first, start with gluten or wheat because these are two major ones.
2. Eliminate this particular food entirely from your diet for a whole month. Make sure you eliminate it in all its forms. For instance, there is gluten in beer and in soy sauce.
3. Try to notice any changes and write them down.
4. After a month, eat a lot of that food with as little else as possible to make sure you're only testing this specific ingredient. For instance, eat one bowl of plain pasta if you're testing wheat. Tune into how you feel both physically and mentally. Write it down.
5. Depending on how you feel after eating it, decide whether to keep this food out of your diet or whether to reintroduce it and move on to the next.

Now that we know what not to eat, there is one more thing that we need to discuss to make the most out of those brain-boosting foods.

CHAPTER TWO
how to eat

I KNOW what you might think: "What do you mean how to eat? I know how to do it! As a matter of fact, I've done it since I was a baby. Just give me the recipes!" I will, but hold back fire, friend. I want to share a few other juicy tips with you. These are all strategies that have helped me a lot, alongside choosing the right brain-boosting foods.

UNPROCESS YOUR DIET

We've already touched on that in the previous chapter, so you know to check the label, and you know what not to buy. So what should you buy? Before we go into more detail about that in the next chapter, as a general rule, you should purchase fresh products you will prepare and cook yourself. Sounds like a lot of work? Don't worry; we'll cover that later. For now, just know this general rule.

When you cook, try to practice 'clean cooking.' In this case, that simply means you don't want to reproduce the unhealthy processing you've just avoided buying at the supermarket. So don't add sugar or aspartame; go easy on the salt, and avoid fat. Actually, not all fat, but more about that later. When I say 'avoid fat,' I mean you want to avoid cooking with fat. So avoid frying unless it is air-frying, and use grilling or steaming instead.

Quality over quantity

There are two things here. First, just because a particular food is healthy doesn't mean you can eat as much as you want of it. Some of the (healthy) foods I will share with you in the next chapter are very high in calories, so I want to make sure you are aware of that. Overeating doesn't help with brain functions. Trust me on that one. I've been there. And you definitely don't want to undereat either for all sorts of reasons, including that you can only fire on all cylinders with enough nutrients.

I'm not asking you to count your calories. Still, if you're not familiar with the energy density of common foods, you might want to track your intake for a while to make sure you're eating enough but not too much. But, of course, how many calories you should eat will vary greatly depending on gender, age, height, physical activity, etc. So I'm inviting you to do your own research. But to give you an idea, an average woman should eat around 2,000 calories per day, and it goes down to 1,800 for women over 50.

So with that in mind, you want to choose your food wisely. It is like spending money: if you have a limited budget, you want to spend your money on things that matter and keep extravagant spending an exception, not a rule. Well, basically, it is the same with food. If eating a chocolate muffin is going to cost you 440 calories and leave you with brain fog for the morning, while a scrambled egg on brown toast is going to cost you 250 calories and will keep you going till lunchtime both physically and mentally, which one do you think you should pick? Yes, let's go with eggs on toast.

Mindful Eating

Another piece of advice I received for managing my ADHD was to try mindfulness. While this is still an ongoing process, and I still really struggle with being 'in the moment,' in the periods when I've managed to stick with it for a few days, I have noticed a difference. Mindfulness is a way of self-calming, so it is pretty evident how it would help anyone with ADHD.

Raise your hand if you like to multitask. That's right, my hand is up too. This is probably a weird way of putting it, but you can look at mindful eating as a way of killing two birds with one stone: it's an opportunity to practice both healthy eating and mindfulness.

Okay, more seriously, what is mindful eating? Simply put, it is focusing on eating while you're eating and not doing anything else. That's right: no watching TV, no reading the newspaper, no texting friends, no scrolling down social media feeds, and definitely no working at your desk.

Besides having a calming effect, mindful eating is meant to help us eat the quantity we need, not less and not more. Studies have shown that if you're doing something else while eating, your brain is not registering the food, causing you to overeat. I also know that a lot of women with ADHD tend to hyperfocus and will forget to eat. Obviously, this is not going to help our cognitive functions either. So, if that's you, put a timer on to remember to take a break, or you could ask someone to have lunch with you. Whatever it is, sit down and have lunch (and all the other meals).

A simple way to practice mindful eating is to engage your senses and ask yourself the following questions:

- How hungry am I?
- How does this food smell?
- How warm/cold is this food?
- How crunchy/smooth is it?
- Is it now smooth enough for me to swallow it?
- What noise does it make when I chew?
- How do I like the taste?
- How satisfying is it?

You can also put your fork down and try to pay attention to the rest of your body and to the world around you. Am I sitting comfortably? And if you're eating in company, do enjoy the company, but still take a few seconds to tune in now and again.

So, I think we're now fully prepared to look at what we should put on that plate. So, without further delay, let me introduce you to all the smart choices we can make to power our brain (and body) and manage ADHD symptoms.

CHAPTER THREE
wholesome to be awesome

NOW WE KNOW the general rules: what to avoid, how to cook clean, and how to choose wisely. Let's take a look at the 101 foods you can eat (and drink) to improve concentration, motivation, mood, and memory.

One of the first wise swaps you can make is to trade refined (processed) grains for whole grains. So, for instance, forget white rice and start using brown rice. There are a couple of reasons for this.

Whole grains have a lot more fiber than refined carbohydrates, and fibers will keep you fuller for longer and help fight ghrelin, also known as the 'hunger hormone.' It also helps balance your blood sugar, and blood sugar is closely tied to mood swings.

Of course, you already know everything about sugar. So similarly, consuming a lot of refined carbohydrates will create a surge in blood sugar, which will trigger a high insulin response and be followed by hypoglycemia. In addition, it can create or worsen symptoms such as irritability, anxiety, and nervousness.

The recommended daily fiber intake for adults is around 25g per day. Most people need to eat more fiber. One easy way to boost that number is to start eating the unrefined version of carbohydrates.

So, are you sold on the idea of eating whole grains? Great! Let me give you some ideas of a few you can try. I have hand-picked the following ones, as they have a higher protein content, and spoiler alert: ADHD brains need protein. I will cover this in-depth in a minute. Admittedly, grains are not big on proteins, but we might as well make this food group work extra hard for us.

So here are some high(er) protein grains you can try. The protein amount is per 100g of food, uncooked.

- Oats, 17g
- Whole wheat pasta, 15g
- Wild rice, 15g
- Buckwheat, 13g
- Quinoa, 13g
- Millet, 11g

This is definitely not an exhaustive list, and you're, of course, welcome to try some other whole grains, such as:

- Whole wheat
- Brown rice
- Barley
- Rye
- Corn (whole grain cornmeal)
- Amaranth
- Farro
- Spelt
- Kamut
- Teff
- Bulgur
- Sorghum

- Freekeh
- Triticale
- Emmer

Not sure you're going to remember all of those before going grocery shopping? I got you covered and created this handy cheat sheet. You can grab it here: bit.ly/brainboostingrecipes

Now, I bet you can't wait to know more about I am starting to make such a fuss about protein, so go on, move to the next chapter.

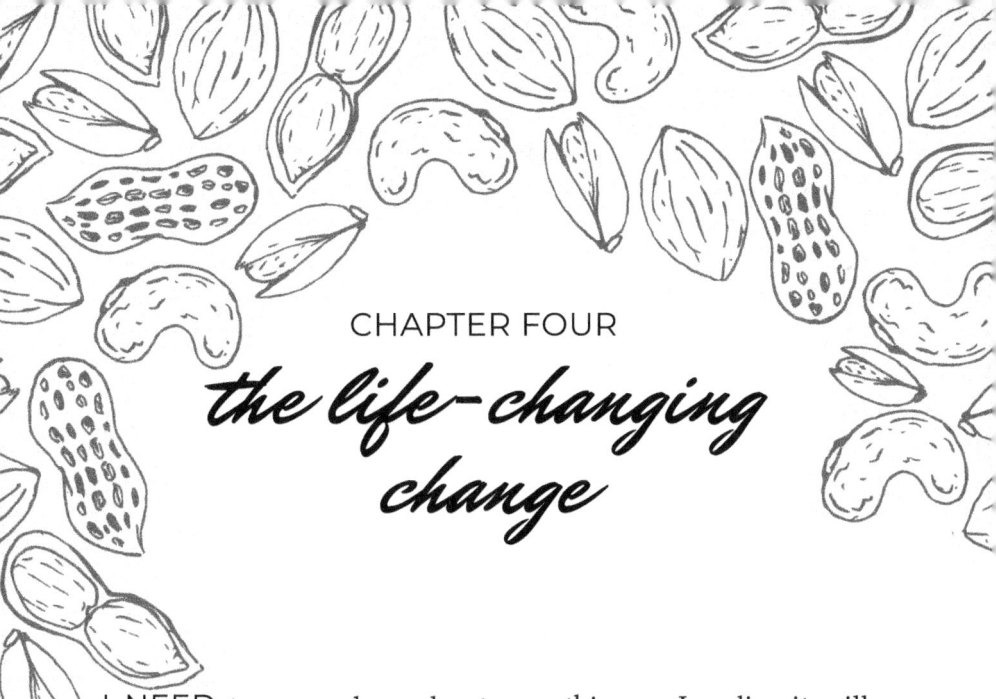

CHAPTER FOUR
the life-changing change

I NEED to come clean about something as I realize it will affect my recommendations: I'm a vegan. I have been eating a plant-based diet for the last six years and wouldn't change it for the world. But it has made my relationship with protein a bit more complicated.

When I went vegan, I completely fell into the narrative that there is no such thing as protein deficiency and that plants will cover your protein needs effortlessly. It's a statement thrown around a lot in vegan circles, including in all the popular documentaries that have inspired many people to reduce their meat and dairy intake. While I understand what they mean when they say that, I have learned the hard way that it is a bit more complicated than it first sounds.

It is one of the reasons you will find a lot of plant-based protein recommendations in this book. Now, if you're vegan or vegetarian yourself, you're welcome; no need to thank me. If you're not, you're welcome too, since the maximum recommended weekly meat intake is 455g cooked. So let's say that covers three to four meals. You're going to need inspiration for what to eat for all of the other meals.

The jury is still out on how much protein people should eat, and you often find calculators using 0.8 grams of protein per kilogram of body weight. But age and amount of exercise are factors too. To give you a vague idea, though, it is around 50g for many people. This may not sound like much, but it requires planning if you're going to eat clean, high-quality protein. By 'clean,' I mean unprocessed and lean. In other words, without the unhealthy fats mostly found in red meat.

My main takeaway on protein and managing ADHD, besides making sure I reach my daily intake, is to ensure that I eat protein throughout the day. This is very important to support executive functions. So make sure you get protein at least three times a day: for breakfast, lunch, and dinner.

Does 'life-changing' sound like an overstatement? It isn't in my case. Working on my protein intake had a huge impact on my cognitive functions. So, where can we find proteins that will power our brains throughout the day?

ANIMAL PRODUCTS

Okay, I think I've made my case against red meat strongly enough. Just one more recommendation: buy the most ethical meat, fish, and eggs you can afford. Not only is it the ethical thing to do, but it is also better for your health. You don't want the antibiotics and hormones these animals have been given to get into your bloodstream, so always try to pick free-range, antibiotic-free, hormone-free, etc.

Now, let's look at what animal products you can eat if you so wish (protein is given per 100g of food) and keep in mind that how you cook them is also important:

Chicken breast (skinless, cooked): 23g.

Pasture-raised chicken has more antioxidants and omega-3 than battery chicken.

Turkey breast (skinless, cooked, roasted): 30g.

Fish and seafood

These are excellent choices in terms of lean protein, but you have to be careful not to eat too much of them because they contain mercury. The current recommendation is no more than three times a week or twice a week for pregnant women. You might want to check www.seafoodwatch.org for recommendations. With that in mind, here are some of the highest-protein fish and seafood:

- Cod: 19g
- Halibut: 23g
- Pollock: 19g
- Shrimp: 23g
- Tilapia 26g
- Tuna 29g

Eggs (whole): 13g

Free-range eggs are an easy and excellent choice of protein for breakfast. Keep some boiled eggs in the fridge and grab one or two if you're in a rush and don't have time to make breakfast. Eggs help your brain much more than a bowl of processed cereal. The white has more protein overall, but the yolk has a lot of other good things that can boost your immune system and lower blood pressure.

PLANT-BASED

As I have already pointed out, you'll need some plant-based protein at some point, even if you're not on a plant-based diet.

Once you've had meat for three meals and fish for another three, there are still a lot of meals left to cover. So, let's look at the plant-based options and see how we can 'pepper' proteins throughout the day.

Processed plant-based protein

The meat replacement options are usually processed, so they're not ideal in our quest to avoid additives. However, there are some processed products worth mentioning. They are only processed in the sense that they have been prepared, but they shouldn't contain too many harmful additives. I use them a lot, as I immediately gave up when I looked at a recipe to make tofu from scratch.

- Firm tofu, 17g: this figure varies a lot, so you should look at the package. The secret to eating tofu is to press it, get rid of the water, and then marinate it to absorb the flavors. Believe it or not, my kids love tofu.
- Silken tofu, 8g: again, it varies a lot, so look at the package. This is my go-to option for breakfast. I blend it with fruits, making a super simple, delicious, and nutritious smoothie.
- Tempeh, 19g: Like tofu, tempeh is made of soybeans. It is a traditional Indonesian food, and it is slightly fermented. You really want to marinate it to enjoy it.
- Seitan, 25g: it is made of wheat gluten, so it is definitely not an option for everyone, but I wanted to give it a mention, as you might come across it in meat-replacement foods. And if you tolerate it, it can be a nice change from tofu.

Nuts and seeds

Nuts and seeds are great as they all contain healthy fat in addition to protein, and that's another thing we're after to support our brain - but more about that later.

The only word of caution with nuts and seeds (besides obvious allergies) is that they have a high-calorie density, so don't go nuts on nuts and seeds (pun intended). To give you an idea, I often carry a tiny container of almonds with me as a snack: it contains 15 almonds, about 100 calories. The other thing is that, like everything else, you want to eat them unprocessed, so no BBQ roasted peanuts, no marmite cashew nuts, no salted pistachios, or other delights. Sorry.

So here are your best options in terms of protein ratio. As usual, the amount of protein is per 100g of food:

- Peanuts, 26g
- Raw almonds, 21g
- Sunflower seeds, 21g
- Pistachios, 20g
- Pumpkin seeds, 19g
- Cassuts, 18g
- Chia seeds, 17g
- Hazelnuts, 15g
- Walnuts, 15g
- Pine nuts, 14g
- Brazil nuts, 14g

Just a few ideas about how to 'sprinkle' nuts and seeds in your diet:

- Add a tablespoon of pumpkin seeds to your smoothie.
- Add ¼ cup of cashews to your stir fry.
- Carry them as part of a snack mix.

Legumes and beans

Legumes and beans are an essential part of my diet, and it's the same for most healthy vegans. But, overall, they are underrepresented in Western cuisine, and that's a shame, given all the benefits they can bring. For our purposes, we're going to focus on protein, but keep in mind that they are also very rich in fiber, which we want to increase too. Having said that, if you're not used to eating a lot of beans, consider introducing them to your diet gradually to be kind to your digestive system.

You can find a lot more than the ones mentioned here. I have selected these because of their higher protein content, and I've indicated the amount of protein per 100g of beans:

- Fava beans (dry), 26g
- Edamame, 18g
- Lupin beans, 16g
- Large white beans, 10g
- Chickpeas, 9g: they are also high in serotonin, which is known as a mood stabilizer that helps regulate attention and emotions.
- Lentils, 9g
- Cranberry beans or borlotti beans, 9g
- Pinto beans, 9g
- Kidney beans, 9g
- Black beans, 9g
- Split peas, 8g
- Navy beans or haricot beans, 8g
- Lima beans or butter beans, 8g

Now, I know that plant-based protein inspiration can be tricky both for both vegans and non-vegans folks alike. That's why I've created a little ebook just for you with all my personal favorite recipes. It's got breakfast, main meals, and snack ideas. And you can get it with all the other freebies I've prepared for you: bit.ly/brainboostingrecipes

And just to hammer it home one last time before we move on to the next chapter: remember to keep your proteins clean and to incorporate them throughout the day for optimal brain function.

CHAPTER FIVE
the unlikely sidekick

FUN FACT: Nearly 70% of our brain is made out of fat, and fat is very important for our brain to function. Now, if you've ever been on a diet (other than keto, I guess), it might be difficult to come to terms with the idea that fat is good for you. So, let's say it 3 times out loud together: Fat is good for me. Fat is good for me. Fat is good for me.

Okay, admittedly, not all fats are made equal, and they're not all good for us. So, let's take a closer look. We've already covered which food to avoid, and that is mostly because they contain the wrong kind of fat. We want to avoid saturated fat, which can be found in some animal products like butter and red meat. And we want to avoid trans fat, which can be found in processed, ready-made foods like baked goods, frozen pizzas, margarine, etc. You also absolutely want to avoid fried food. Sorry.

But there are all sorts of good-fat foods out there, and the ones we're particularly after contain omega 3. So here are plenty of ideas of what you can eat to boost your healthy fat intake and boost your brain as a result.

Animal Products

Fish

Fish are best known for their high content of omega-3, and they are the first food to be mentioned if you start to look for healthy fat. The top contenders are:

- Salmon
- Anchovies
- Halibut
- Sardines

But, as we've mentioned, it is not recommended to eat fish more than three times a week, so you're going to need to add other sources to properly up the amount of healthy fat in your diet.

Lamb

Lamb is the only meat that is high in omega 3, so let's take a look at some plant-based options we can add to boost our brains.

Plant-Based

Nuts and seeds

Nuts and seeds are an excellent source of healthy fat, and they also contain fiber, which, as we've seen earlier, will help us stay fuller for longer and stabilize our mood. But nuts and seeds are also very high in calories, as mentioned in the protein section, so if you're not used to them, take your food scale out the first few times you're introducing them to your diet and make sure you're getting the right amount.

On top of healthy fats, some nuts and seeds also have added benefits for people with ADHD:

- Antioxidants prevent cognitive decline. They are mostly known as Vitamin C, Vitamin E, and beta carotene.
- Zinc, also an antioxidant, helps with concentration and blood sugar levels.
- Magnesium helps with sleep and reduces stress.
- Thiamine (or B1) keeps the nervous system healthy.
- Selenium, another antioxidant, helps prevent mental decline.
- As we know, fiber helps regulate blood sugar, which helps with mood swings.
- Calcium regulates neurotransmitters.

So, here are my top picks for healthy fats with added benefits:

- Almonds also have reasonable amounts of protein and antioxidants.
- Brazil nuts contain zinc, magnesium, thiamine (or B1), selenium, and fiber.
- Cashews contain magnesium, zinc, and antioxidants.
- Coconut is high in medium-chain triglycerides, which help with brain tissue.
- Hemp seeds have a good amount of protein.
- Sesame seeds contain calcium and zinc.
- Walnuts have the most omega-3. They also contain antioxidants, vitamin E, selenium, and magnesium.

Fruits and Vegetables

Fruits and vegetables are not particularly famous for containing fat, but here are a few worth mentioning:

- Acai berries
- Avocado
- Maca root
- Seaweed: that's where the fish get their omega-3 from, so it's an excellent option for vegetarians.
- Leafy greens contain omega 3. Although it is not a huge amount, the following are worth a mention:
- Kale contains iron, which can help with fatigue.
- Spinach contains iron, too.
- Romaine lettuce
- Arugula
- Purslane

Oils

Who would have thought?! I kept the most obvious for last. Here are my top three:

- Olive oil
- Coconut oil
- Grapeseed oil

But remember that how you use oil is important. We're not talking about frying food here. We're only talking about the benefits of eating oil at room temperature.

There you go. That was 24 food items to choose from to boost your brain with healthy fat. But if you're struggling to include them in your diet or if you can't feel any obvious benefits, you can find omega-3 supplements in health stores. Most of them are made of fish oil, but you can find vegetarian versions easily. Of course, you need to check with your doctor first, but it might be worth looking into.

CHAPTER SIX
no beauty without color

COLORFUL FRUITS and vegetables are where antioxidants live. They also all have fiber, and that's why we need them to complement our protein and healthy fats diet.

Fruits

Besides antioxidants, I will mention a few other exciting benefits we might come across when talking about fruits and vegetables:

- Potassium is involved in nerve functions.
- Folate improves cognitive function.
- B2 maintains the body's energy supply.
- B6 is essential in brain development and in keeping a healthy nervous system.
- B12 deficiency can lead to fatigue, depression, and difficulty concentrating. Finding B12 outside of animal products is challenging, so people often take a supplement.

- Vitamin C is an antioxidant and also stabilizes blood sugar.

So here are a few ideas of fruits of great fruits to try, all low in sugar:

- Apples: you know what they say, "An apple a day keeps the doctor away."
- Avocado: also contains potassium and folate.
- Grapefruit
- Pomegranate
- Berries:
- Acai berries contain omega-3
- Blueberries are nicknamed 'brain berries'
- Blackberries
- Cherries
- Goldenberries are a high-protein fruit with 16g for 100g of food. They also contain B1, B2, B6, and B12.
- Goji berries contain vitamin C.

Vegetables

Now, I've selected a few vegetables to add to your rainbow with some added benefits:

- Asparagus
- Bell peppers contain vitamin C.
- Beets contain folate and beta-carotene.
- Broccoli
- Brussels sprouts
- Cabbage
- Cauliflower
- Chlorella is meant to detoxify, particularly mercury, so it's good to eat in combination with fish.

- Horseradish contains calcium, potassium, and vitamin C.
- Leeks
- Onions
- Spirulina has an incredibly high ratio of protein. It also contains iron.
- Sweet potatoes
- Yellow squash

As I've mentioned with animal products before, how food is produced matters. As such, if you can afford to buy organic, it is better for your health to avoid eating pesticides. At the very least, here are the so-called dirty dozen, the 12 fruits and vegetables that consistently carry a higher level of pesticides:

- Strawberries
- Apples
- Nectarines
- Peaches
- Celery
- Grapes
- Cherries
- Spinach
- Tomatoes
- Sweet bell peppers
- Cherry tomatoes
- Cucumbers

On the other hand, here are the clean 15: the 15 fruits and vegetables that have lower pesticide residues and so are more okay to buy non-organic:

- Avocados
- Sweet Corn
- Pineapples
- Cabbage
- Sweet peas (frozen)

- Onions
- Asparagus
- Mangos
- Papayas
- Kiwi
- Eggplant
- Honeydew melon
- Grapefruit
- Cantaloupe
- Cauliflower

Whoa, that's a lot of fruits and vegetables to choose from! Don't worry; they're all in a handy cheat sheet, and you can download it here: bit.ly/brainboostingrecipes

Are you scared you're going to turn into a rabbit now? Don't be. Just glancing at the free cookbook I've added should reassure you, but I also want to introduce you to a lovely treat in the next chapter.

CHAPTER SEVEN
the helpful treat

TREATS

I COULD HAVE INCLUDED dark chocolate in the beans section, but its benefits don't include protein. However, raw cocoa beans can stimulate serotonin and endorphins, which make us happy. Besides, they contain the following:

- Antioxidants
- Flavonoids that increase blood flow
- Magnesium
- Iron
- Chromium, which regulates blood sugar level
- Zinc
- Copper, which keeps nerve cells healthy

So, to be able to keep all those wonderful properties, you want to try to consume chocolate as unprocessed as possible, like everything else: so definitely dark and raw if possible. Enjoy! Obviously, you have to keep moderation in mind, but 'Peanut Butter and Chocolate Mousse' for breakfast is totally an option! In fact, it's more than that: it's in the four-week meal plan I've devised for you, and you'll find the recipe in the cookbook.

Herbs

Another kind of treat is to spice things up a little. 'Clean cooking' doesn't have to be bland, and we might as well use spices that will benefit us.

Here are a few that are worth a mention:

- Saffron is a proven anti-depressant.
- Cinnamon helps with blood sugar levels and attention and is an antioxidant.
- Garlic boosts blood flow to the brain.
- Oregano also increases blood flow to the brain.
- Rosemary is known in folk culture to help with memory. As Shakespeare's Ophelia says, "There's rosemary, that's for remembrance." Several studies have now proven its beneficial effects on memory and concentration.
- Thyme is also proven to help with memory.
- Sage is another one that helps with memory.

You can now see how some organic vegetables with a bit of olive oil and one of those herbs could be kind to your brain and taste delicious at the same time. Sometimes, simple is best.

CHAPTER EIGHT
what to drink

I WANTED to include a short section on drinks, as they are another thing we ingest, and, as a result, they impact our brains.

Water

This one sounds pretty obvious. Of course, we need water. I know. You know. And I know you know. The only reason I'm including it here is to put a little reminder to drink water regularly throughout the day. Who here can hyperfocus and forget to drink for hours? Me! And that's a guaranteed brain fog for the rest of the day. So, like with protein, it's not just about hitting the 1.5-2L recommended daily intake; it's about spreading it throughout the day.

I've got a couple of tricks that help me. One is to have a water bottle with me while I'm working. It helps me remember to drink because it is right there, and that is easier than breaking the flow to go to the kitchen to fill a glass. The other trick, and this one's more relevant if you live in a country with cold winters, is to drink hot water. I have realized I crave warm drinks when it's cold, but they don't need to be flavored.

Coffee

I hesitated to include coffee in this list. The jury is still out on that one. I've read research saying that it is beneficial for people with ADHD and helps with focus, but there is also a lot of advice that says not to drink coffee because of certain side effects. The most obvious of these is that it can disturb sleep, and that's definitely not a good thing.

I have a long love story with coffee, a slightly toxic one, actually. I've tried to leave a few times but always return. My way of managing the side effects is that even though I drink too much of it, I stop drinking it at lunchtime, hoping it won't keep me up at night.

Another major drawback of coffee is that it prevents iron absorption, and, as a vegan, I want to absorb all the iron I can with my meals.

So, let's take a look at some alternatives to coffee.

Green Tea

Green tea can be a great alternative to coffee. It contains a lot of antioxidants and has the metabolism-boosting EGCG that some of us enjoy in coffee, but it also contains theanine, which helps relax and focus simultaneously. What's not to like?

Herbal teas

In the same way that it's nice to bring some flavor with a purpose to our cooking with the help of herbs, we can bring flavor with a purpose to our water. This is where herbal teas come in. There are a lot to choose from, so I've decided to focus only on the ones that are easy to buy and don't require finding a special herbalist's shop.

Some of the herbs we've mentioned above for cooking are very nice as herbal teas as well. Rosemary and sage, which are both good for memory and concentration, can be made into tea. Rosemary has the added benefit of lifting the mood a little, too. I really like the taste of both, and I often drink them in the afternoon.

My personal favorite for managing ADHD is lemon balm, another easily available tea. Like rosemary and sage, it is good for boosting memory and concentration, but it also helps fight against anxiety and nervousness. As a result, I tend to drink it in the evening, often mixed with other relaxing teas.

Chamomile and lavender are my go-to relaxing herbs, and I often mix them with lemon balm. Although they're not specifically recommended for people with ADHD, I find they're just good all-rounders, calming and comforting teas to drink in the evening to start to wind down.

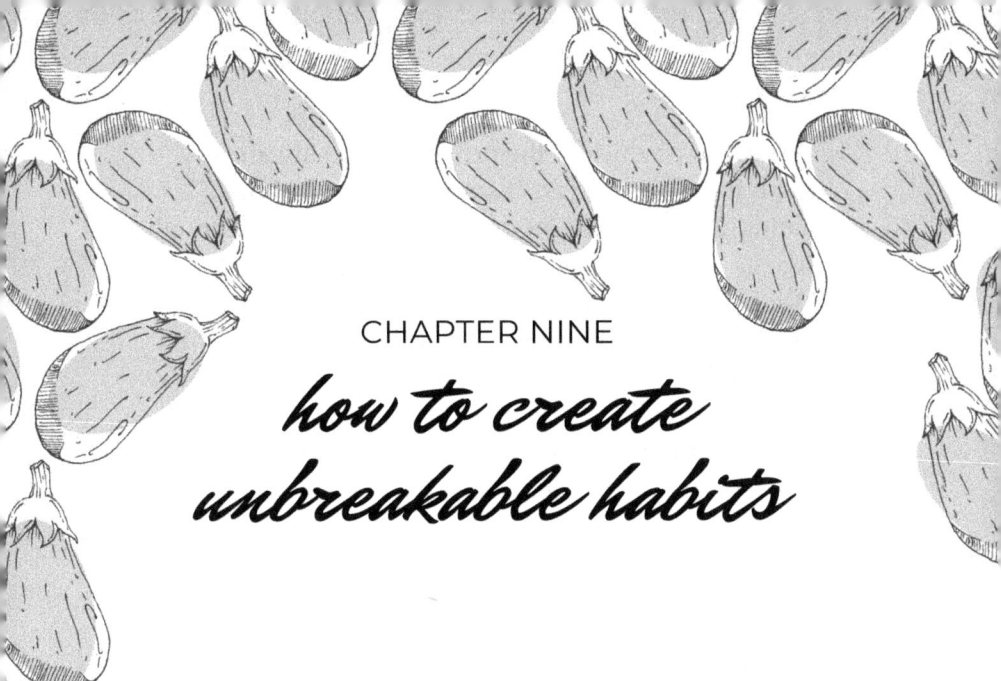

CHAPTER NINE
how to create unbreakable habits

CONGRATULATIONS ON MAKING it all the way here! We're nearly at the end, and I realize this might be a lot to take in in one go. You might be thinking, "But I can't do all that, my eating can't be *that* 'clean,' *that* 'virtuous.'" You're right. And mine is not, don't worry. But I just try to apply most of the principles, most of the time, in a perfectly imperfect manner.

We're in it for the long haul. Our ADHD is not going anywhere, so supporting our brain with lifestyle changes is not like a fad diet that we're going to be obsessed with for a few months and then forget all about it once it starts to work.

Rules

Create your own rules

Grab a paper and a pen, and let's create our own rules:

1. Write down which of the principles you are already applying. For me, it is: "I am quite careful about eating protein throughout the day and getting enough omega 3."
2. Write down which principles you could start applying right now. For instance, in my case, it is "I want to buy more organic fruits and vegetables."
3. Write down which principles you would like to start applying in the future. In my case, "I would like to wean myself off coffee."

Break the rules

That's right. Let's break those brand-new rules. Let's say you're invited to a birthday party, and you are trying to avoid sugar. Never mind, have some cake. But make use of it: take it as an experience. First, be present for every single bite: is it nice? Is it actually worth it? Make a note - a mental note, or even take your phone out and write it down. Then try to notice any changes: are you feeling more wired than without sugar? Are you finding it harder to sleep that night? Are you fuller when dinner comes and don't eat as much in the evening?

Find some opportunities to conduct those controlled experiments. Now, don't get me wrong, I'm not saying break all the rules all the time. I'm not saying have some cake at any single opportunity. I've found that with time, I have developed the ability to decide whether breaking my rules is worth it or not.

Replace rules with intentions

Remember our friend mindfulness? Well, there is another way of practicing mindfulness, and it is to set an intention. So instead of having a rigid rule that says, "I mustn't do that," you set an intention in the morning to behave in a certain way. If we keep the sugar example, that will be "I'm setting the intention not to have any sugar today," and then you become a non-judgemental observer of your day.

Easier said than done, I know. But give it a go. It might help make it a life habit.

Tailor it to your life

If you live a very quiet life on your own, then great! You will probably have a lot of time to implement these ideas and test which ones work best for you. But if you live in the real world, chances are that there are quite a few things that might get in the way, so here are a couple of tips:

Control the meals you can

We're not in an all-or-nothing situation. We're simply trying to implement lifestyle changes. So, some omega 3 is better than none, proteins for breakfast and lunch are better than just for lunch, etc.

If you live with other people and you feel that you can't impose your changes on everyone, control what you can. Start with breakfast, maybe. It's not unusual for people to eat different things for breakfast. If you work or if you have children who go to school, you might be able to plan your own lunch. So that's already two out of the three main meals. If those two are filled with lean protein, healthy fat, whole grains, and a lot of colorful fruits and vegetables, I bet you will start feeling an improvement in your concentration and mood pretty soon.

Plan

But there is just never enough time! I hear you. I realize it may sound boring, but the only way for me to make sure I eat healthily is to plan. I plan weekly, and I plan daily. That's why I've included a blank meal plan in your downloadable pack. You can get it at: bit.ly/brainboostingrecipes

Over the weekend, I write the meal plan for the week along with a shopping list to make sure I will have everything I need. I don't like doing it, but what I do like is not having to think about it for the rest of the week: I simply have to read the plan, and I know what to cook and eat.

Then, every night, I have an auto-reminder that says "prep food," and that's just to make sure that I prepare my lunch for the next day before I crash. When I say "prepare," I don't mean it has to be anything fancy. Most of the time, it means putting what I've just had for dinner in a Tupperware. But if I don't do that, I'm likely to get something ready-made from the supermarket, and that's not going to help my concentration or my mood.

That means I batch cook, meaning that I simply cook more than what we're going to eat in the evening. There are four of us, and I usually cook enough for five or six, so there is some left for my next day's lunch, or I freeze a portion for another day.

Another trick to avoid buying processed food is to keep snacks with you. I've included some yummy and healthy snack recipes in the downloadable cookbook. But I can't be bothered to prepare a few healthy treats; as I've mentioned earlier, I often take 15 almonds with me. I like doing that because they don't take any space, and I know that they are full of protein and omega-3. I also often carry an apple in my bag. It is easy to eat anywhere, and it doesn't get bruised easily.

I hope these few tips will help you put all the information I've shared with you into action. To help you do so, I've created a sample meal plan, and I'm going to tell you all about it, just about now.

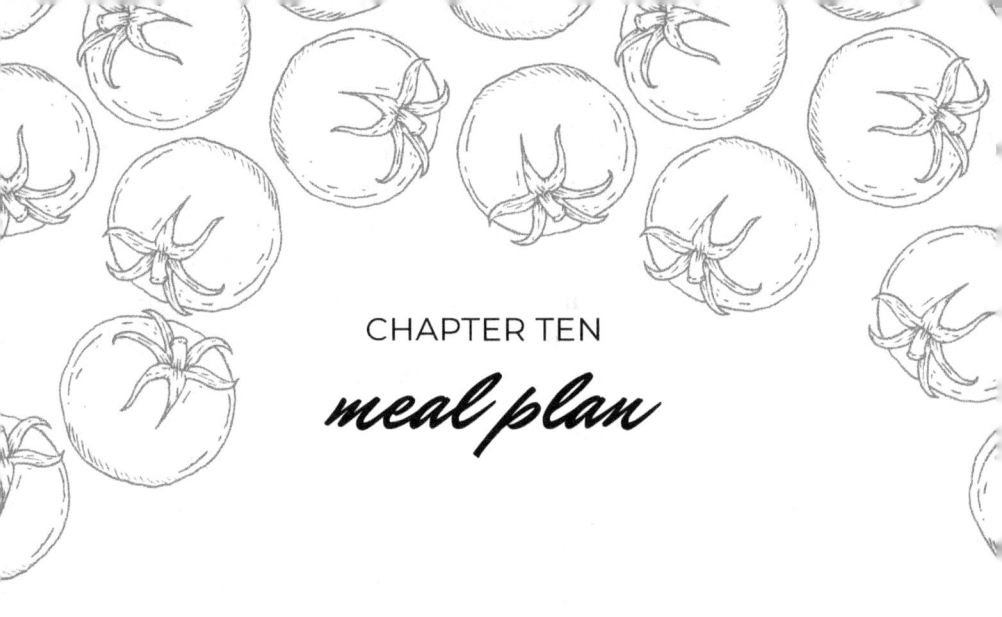

CHAPTER TEN

meal plan

DID you skip straight here in the hope that you can just follow my plan? I would encourage you to rewind and read the rest of the book first. Understanding the principles that underpin this plan is the secret to a life-long change.

I've created this four-week meal plan to give you an idea of what implementing this diet looks like. If you want to follow it to the letter, you can, but this is intended as an example and inspiration to create a plan tailored to your life circumstances and tastes. So, if you haven't done it yet, download the blank meal plan and use it to draft what *your* plan will look like. Do you need the link again? I've got you covered: bit.ly/brainboostingrecipes

Now, let's look at the plan together and how you might want to customize it.

There are a few assumptions in this plan. One of them is that you have more time to cook on Saturday and Sunday. Over the weekend, I have scheduled making healthy treats to eat the following week and slightly more hearty dinners to batch cook and keep for lunch later. If that doesn't suit your life, you can start by reshuffling that on your blank plan.

You will notice that I have also scheduled some batch cooking on weekday evenings. When I say "batch cooking," I simply mean cooking one or two extra portions. Then, I scheduled the same dish a couple of days later. The idea is to make it short enough to keep in the fridge but leave a little gap to make it more exciting. If you find it confusing and would rather eat it the next day, go ahead and do that.

I have only included main courses as I don't need to patronize you by suggesting a fruit for dessert and a side salad if you feel like it. It is not intended to restrict you to a main course only as long as it is in keeping with the guidelines we've discussed, you are, of course, welcome to add to this base.

Talking of base, many dishes are customizable, and in your free recipe book, I have included five different variations for meals, like shakes, stir-fry, and hummus. Again, this is just to get you started, and you can create your own.

Are you getting hungry just by looking at snack recipes like the 'Protein Muffin,' but you don't usually eat snacks? Don't worry, friend. Who said they had to be eaten as a snack? Not me! Eat them as breakfast or a dessert with a lighter main course like the Ceasar Salad. Same thing with the 'longer' breakfast recipes: Do you like the sound of them but can't cook and won't cook in the morning? Eat them for lunch! In short, it is your plan, and you make it work for you.

The meals in this plan have been selected on three grounds: they're high in plant-based protein, high in omega 3, and can be prepared in 15 minutes or under.

Why high in protein and omega 3? You know why by now. And if you don't, you can revisit chapters 4 and 5.

Why plant-based? It's not (just) because I want to convert you; it is because this is the inspiration most people need when eating lean proteins. And that's why I'm giving you a free recipe book where you will find all the recipes for the dishes you will see here. You don't need me to eat a chicken breast or two eggs. So, it goes without saying that if you eat animal products, you can add them to your plan. Just remember that we can all benefit from eating more plant-based proteins.

Why 15 minutes? To make sure being time short is not an excuse, and I know we're living in a world where time is always short.

So grab your blank plan and pen and create your own plan. If planning four weeks in one go feels overwhelming, just make one week at a time. Then, by the end of the month, you will have your very own four-week meal plan that you can repeat indefinitely.

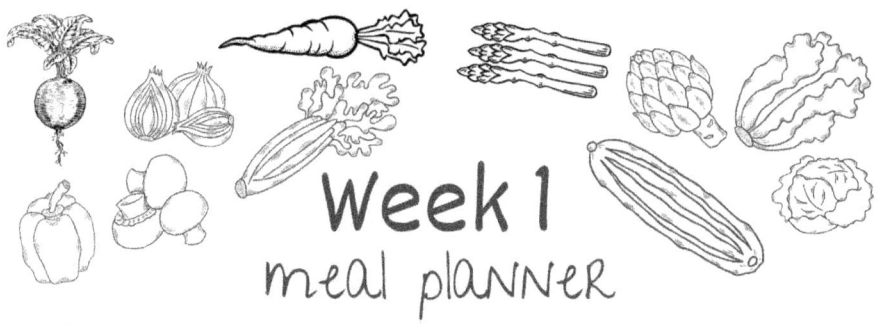

Week 1 meal planner

	BREAKFAST	LUNCH	DINNER	SNACKS
M	FLAXSEED OATMEAL WITH FRUIT AND NUTS	HUMMUS WRAP	SZECHUAN TOFU STIR-FRY WITH QUINOA	PROTEIN MUFFIN
T	PEANUT BUTTER AND CHOCOLATE MOUSSE	CHICKPEA SALAD WITH AVOCADO	SPICY PEANUT NOODLES	HUMMUS WITH CARROTS AND CELERY STICKS
W	TROPICAL PARADISE PROTEIN PUNCH	SWEET AND SOUR TOFU STIR-FRY WITH QUINOA	LENTIL SOUP	ROASTED CHICKPEAS
T	CHIA SEED PUDDING WITH COCA NIBS AND NUT BUTTER	HIGH-PROTEIN SNACK PLATE	MEDITERREANEAN PASTA	TRAIL MIX WITH NUTS AND SEEDS
F	PROTEIN SHAKE WITH PEANUT BUTTER AND BANANA	LENTIL SOUP	BLACK BEAN AND SWEET POTATO TACOS	HUMMUS WITH CARROTS AND CELERY STICKS
S	VEGAN OMLET	QUINOA BOWL	QUINOA SALAD WITH EDAMAME	PROTEIN BALLS
S	PROTEIN PANCAKES	MEDITERRANEAN FLAT BREAD	BBQ JACKFRUIT AND LENTIL SANDWICH	ROASTED TOFU BITES

© Estelle Rose — https://mybook.to/brainboostingfood

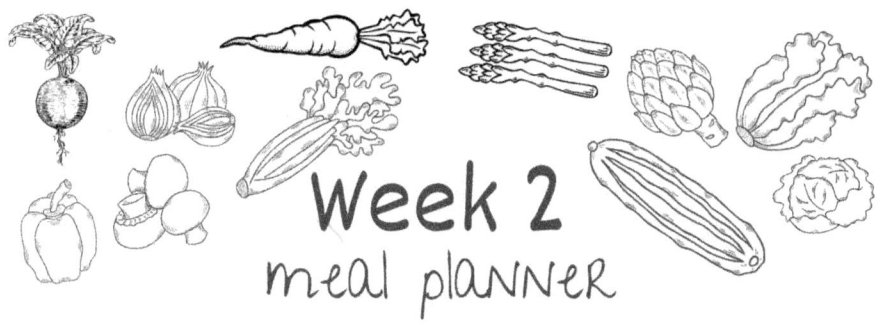

Week 2 meal planner

	BREAKFAST	LUNCH	DINNER	SNACKS
M	GREEN MACHINE PROTEIN SMOOTHIE	QUINOA SALAD WITH EDAMAME	SPICY PEANUT NOODLES	PROTEIN BALLS
T	CHIA SEED PUDDING WITH RAISINS AND CINNAMON	POWER BOWL	VEGAN CAESAR SALAD	ROASTED TOFU BITES
W	FLAXSEED OATMEAL WITH COCOA NIBS AND NUT BUTTER	SPICY PEANUT NOODLES	TERIYAKI STIR-FRY WITH BROWN RICE	TRAIL MIX WITH NUTS AND SEEDS
T	BERRY BLAST PROTEIN	VEGAN CAESAR WRAP	WALNUT AND LENTIL SALAD	PROTEIN BALLS
F	PEANUT BUTTER AND BANANA TOAST	SWEET AND SOUR STIR-FRY WITH BROWN RICE	VEGAN SUSHI BOWL WITH AVOCADO	HUMMUS WITH CARROTS AND CELERY STICKS
S	TOFU SCRAMBLE	HIGH-PROTEIN SNACK PLATE	QUINOA SALAD WITH EDAMAME	BEAN DIP WITH VEGGIE STICKS
S	AVOCADO TOAST WITH HEMP SEED	VEGAN SUSHI BOWL WITH AVOCADO	MOCK DUCK BUTTER BEAN STEW	PROTEIN MUFFIN

© Estelle Rose - https://mybook.to/brainboostingfood

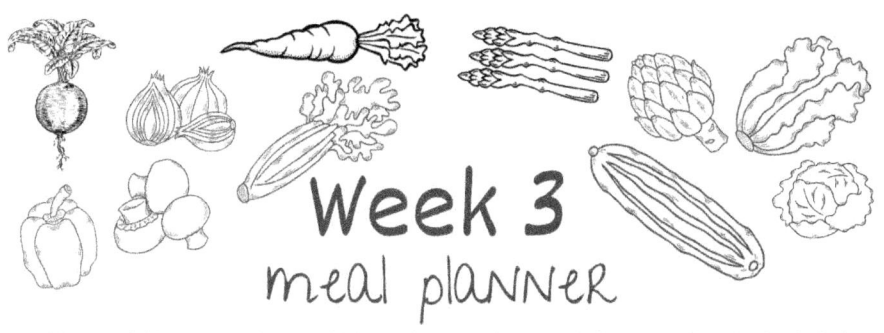

Week 3 meal planner

	BREAKFAST	LUNCH	DINNER	SNACKS
M	CHOCOLATE PROTEIN DELIGHT	HUMMUS WRAP	HEMP SEED PESTO PASTA	BEAN DIP WITH VEGGIE STICKS
T	FLAXSEED OATMEAL WITH COCOA POWDER AND COCONUT FLAKES	MOCK DUCK BUTTER BEAN STEW	POWER BOWL	PROTEIN MUFFIN
W	PEANUT BUTTER AND CHOCOLATE MOUSSE	POWER BOWL	CLASSIC STIR-FRY WITH NOODLES	BEAN DIP WITH VEGGIE STICKS
T	ALMOND BUTTER AND APPLE DELIGHT	HEMP SEED PESTO PASTA	WALNUT AND LENTIL SALAD	TRAIL MIX WITH NUTS AND SEEDS
F	MOCHA MADNESS PROTEIN SHAKE	PEANUT SATAY STIR-FRY WITH NOODLES	VEGAN CAESAR SALAD	HUMMUS WITH CARROTS AND CELERY STICKS
S	PROTEIN PANCAKES WITH BERRIES	BBQ TOFU SANDWICH	MEDITERREANEAN PASTA	PEANUT BUTTER AND CHOCOLATE MOUSSE
S	VEGAN OMLET	VEGAN CAESAR WRAP	SWEET POTATO AND LENTIL CURRY	ROASTED CHICKPEAS

© Estelle Rose – https://mybook.to/brainboostingfood

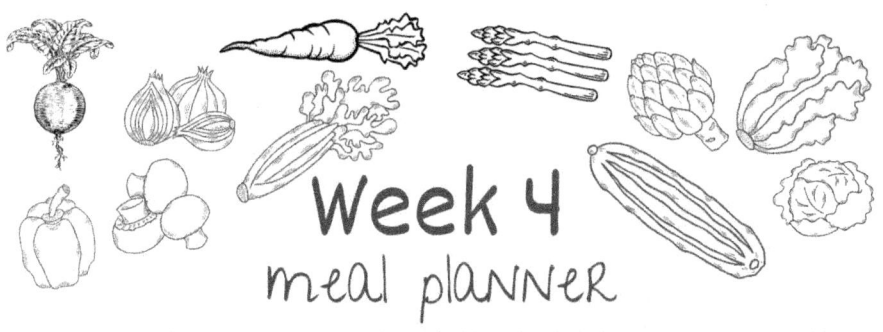

Week 4 meal planner

	BREAKFAST	LUNCH	DINNER	SNACKS
M	PEANUT BUTTER AND BANANA PROTEIN SHAKE	MEDITERRANEAN FLAT BREAD	CHICKPEA SALAD	PEANUT BUTTER AND CHOCOLATE MOUSSE
T	CHIA SEED PUDDING WITH COCOA POWDER AND BERRIES	SWEET POTATO AND LENTIL CURRY	SPICY PEANUT NOODLES	ROASTED CHICKPEAS
W	DATE DREAM TPAST	CHICKPEA SALAD	SZECHUAN STIR-FRY WITH BROWN RICE	PEANUT BUTTER AND CHOCOLATE MOUSSE
T	GREEN MACHINE PROTEIN SMOOTHIE	SPICY PEANUT NOODLES	WALNUT AND LENTIL SALAD	HUMMUS WITH CARROTS AND CELERY STICKS
F	FLAXSEED OATMEAL WITH BERRIES AND COCONUT FLAKES	SWEET AND SOUR STIR-FRY WITH BROWN RICE	VEGAN SUSHI BOWL WITH AVOCADO	TRAIL MIX WITH NUTS AND SEEDS
S	AVOCADO TOAST WITH HEMP SEEDS	BBQ TOFU SANDWICH	SWEET POTATO AND BLACK BEAN TACOS	PROTEIN BALLS
S	SWEET POTATOES HASH	HIGH-PROTEIN SNACK PLATE	QUINOA SALAD WITH EDAMAME	VEGAN PROTEIN MUFFIN

© Estelle Rose – https://mybook.to/brainboostingfood

conclusion

You're still reading! That's great, and I'm flattered. I genuinely hope that this was helpful. Changing my diet has helped me so much that I felt compelled to share.

For me, the biggest change came from making sure I get enough protein for each meal and from increasing my healthy fat intake. I also benefited a lot from identifying that wheat isn't my friend, and I try to avoid it when I can, at least the white, refined version. Unprocessing my diet and cooking from scratch is just part of an overall healthy diet, and as a parent and a vegan, I was already trying to do that, so that part wasn't too much of a leap.

What was a huge learning curve in my case was not just what, but how to eat. I now look at what I eat as an imperfect process but one that I am committed to improving over time: Not to beat myself up but to look after myself in the simplest of ways.

So, I encourage you to pick a few things you're willing to try. Conduct your own experiments and see if anything helps improve your concentration, motivation, mood, and memory.

And then share! If you've discovered something that works for you, share it with the world. You can make such a difference in someone's life with just a few words. I'm obviously biased, but one super easy way for you to do that is to leave a review for this book on Amazon. The impact can be huge. Imagine inspiring someone to take a few simple steps towards improving their cognitive function. How cool would that be?

Does the thought of leaving a review overwhelm you? Don't fret. It's super easy, and you can do it in under three minutes. You don't have to write an essay. Just go to the book page (I've even included a QR code), scroll down to "write a customer review," and add a sentence or two. Here are a few prompts to get your creative juice flowing:

- What is your primary learning point from the book? Did you get any aha moment?
- Which of the suggestions are you planning to put into practice? Have you noticed an improvement already?
- How did reading the book make you feel? Hopeful? Empowered?

And boom! Just like that, you've helped someone else in their way to managing their ADHD symptoms. And you've helped me, too. You've helped me reach a larger audience; I am so incredibly grateful for that.

With bottomless energy and boundless gratitude,

Estelle Rose

how to leave a review

So, are you ready to share some brain-boosting love with other women with ADHD and support them on their journey towards thriving?

Leaving a review on Amazon is as easy as 1-2-3:

1. Visit the book's page on Amazon.
2. Scroll down to the "Customer Reviews" section.
3. Click on the "Write a customer review" button.

Once you're there, pour your heart out as if you were talking to a friend. Here are some ideas to get you started:

- Share your insights and favorite parts of the book.
- Describe how the book has made a difference in your life.
- Describe the tone of the book and what makes it unique.

Feel free to get creative! Images speak louder than words sometimes, so add a photo or video to complement your review and make it more personal.

To leave a review, please visit mybook.to/brainboostingfood

You can also scan the QR code below to go directly to the review page.

Sharing love and inspiration triggers an inimitable warm and fuzzy feeling inside and lifts everyone around you. It's the next best thing after coffee ;-)

Seriously though, your authentic words have the pow

er to set someone on their transformative journey towards thriving with ADHD by sparking that sense of hope. Use your power.

Thank you so much for being an essential part of this journey.

SPECIAL GIFTS FOR YOU

GRAB THEM NOW

Follow this link:
bit.ly/brainboostingrecipes

Or scan the QR code

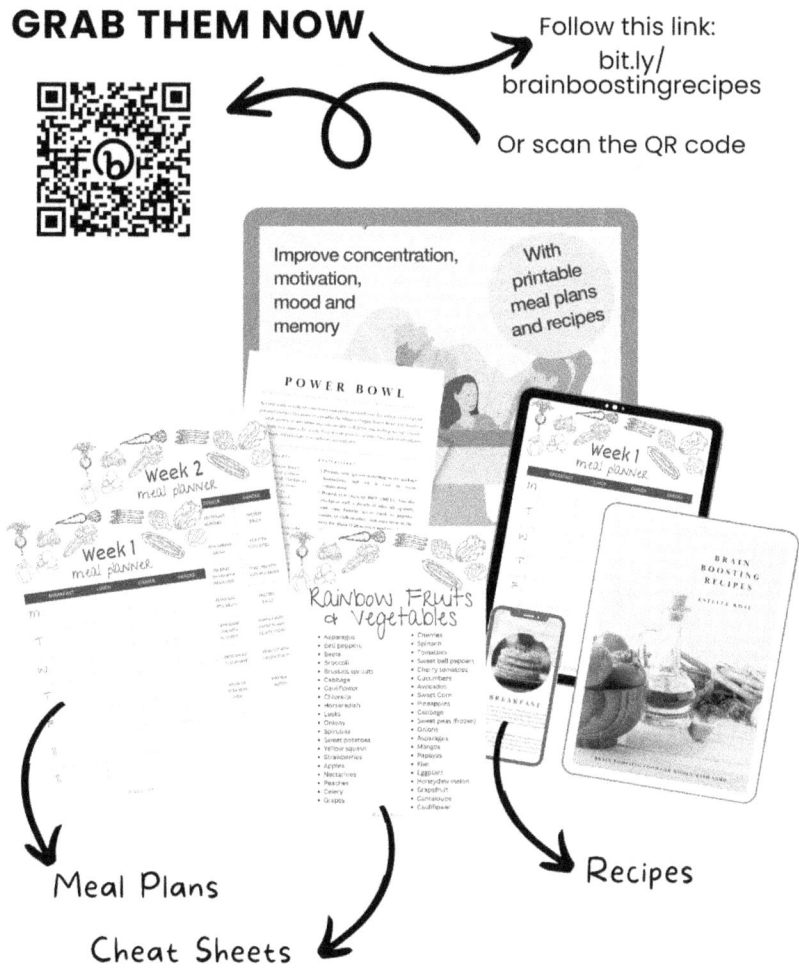

Meal Plans

Cheat Sheets

Recipes

Print or use them with any PDF Annotation App

about the author

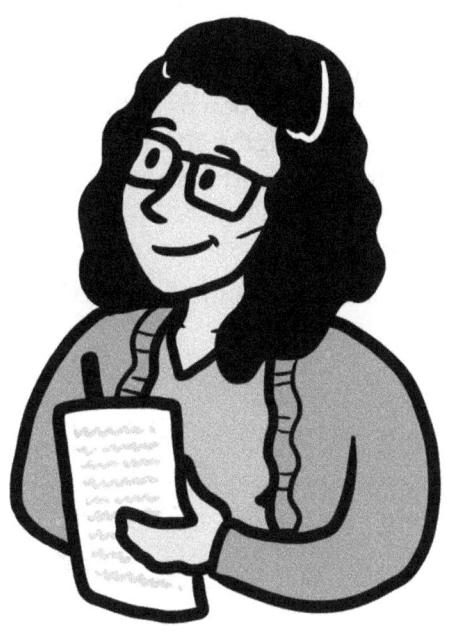

Estelle Rose, author of Empowered Women with ADHD and Brain-Boosting Food for Women with ADHD, is dedicated to helping women with ADHD thrive.

Her guides provide practical strategies for managing symptoms and achieving goals. With a late diagnosis, Estelle understands the unique challenges of ADHD.

She explored psychology, therapies, neuroscience, self-hypnosis, meditation, nutrition, and coaching, gaining valuable insights to manage her own ADHD. This transformative experience fueled her desire to share her experiences and expertise with others.

Estelle's writing is compassionate, insightful, and informative, offering practical tips and strategies. Her warm and engaging style provides invaluable resources for women at all stages of their ADHD journey.

Estelle's commitment to empowering women with ADHD shines through, helping women with ADHD thrive and embrace their unique strengths and making her books essential for those newly diagnosed or who have been living with the condition for years.

instagram.com/rosalipublishing

also by estelle rose

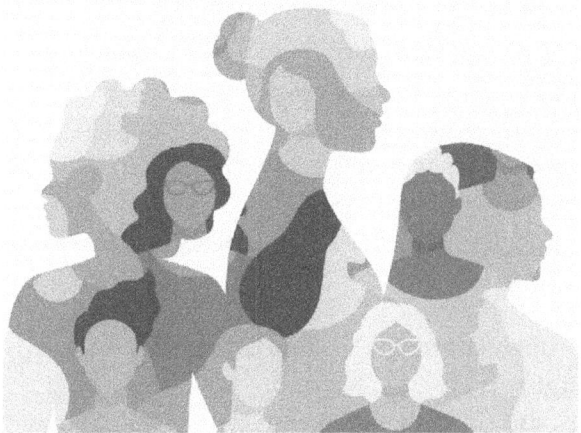

Are you overwhelmed by a million racing thoughts and a never-ending rollercoaster of emotions? Then keep reading.

Do you constantly feel on the edge of burning out? Like you're always either stuck in hyperfocus or hyper-fatigue?

Do you feel held back at work or in relationships? Do you live in constant fear of rejection, criticism, or judgment?

Do you feel like putting your house in order is as big of a task as climbing Mount Everest, even though the clutter around you makes your mind feel cluttered too?

Have you always felt like you didn't quite fit in?

I know. I've been there.

Imagine having a switch to silence the constant chatter in your brain. Imagine feeling accepted and understood for who you truly are.

Did you know that only 3.2% of women in the U.S. are diagnosed with ADHD compared to 5.4% of men? That's 69% more diagnoses for men when the prevalence is about the same!

We've been unseen for far too long. But the tide is turning, and adult women are now the fastest-growing group diagnosed with ADHD.

Inside this complete guide, specifically tailored for women, you'll find a treasure trove of practical tools, hacks, and proven strategies to help you manage your ADHD symptoms.

But you don't just want to survive with ADHD; you want to thrive, right?

With the guidance of this book, you'll learn to make peace with ADHD and embrace neurodiversity to unlock your full potential and live with clarity and confidence.

Here are just a few of the transformative tools and strategies you will discover in this book:

- **15 proven strategies to slow down your racing thoughts** p. 55
- Facts and fiction when it comes to ADHD and women p. 3
- The mindset shift you need to **embrace neurodiversity** p. 15
- The 7-step guide to **regulating emotions** p. 81
- How to craft your own sensory diet to **address sensory problems** p. 52
- How to **manage your hormones** and their impact on ADHD. p. 8

- The three simple steps you need to tackle the floordrobe (you know, that pile of clothes on the floor). And many more hacks to **create a calming home**. p. 96
- How to make peace with your bank account and **curb emotional spending** p. 123
- The 3-step formula you need to set healthy boundaries p. 138
- How to **navigate your relationships** with friends, family, and professionals. We'll even talk about sex, baby! p. 143
- All the tools to **harness the power of ADHD at work** and tackle impostor syndrome p. 108

And much more!

From the American Psychiatry Association to the Royal College of Psychiatrists in the U.K., leading psychiatric associations emphasize that lifestyle changes can improve ADHD symptoms, with or without medication.

If you're ready to make ADHD work for you rather than against you, then "Empowered Women with ADHD" is the book you need, even if you have the attention span of a goldfish and feel like you're drowning in a sea of information.

It is a practical guide **written by a woman with ADHD for busy women with ADHD. You can start implementing strategies right now and at your own pace.**

So if you want to live your life to your full potential, **get your copy at** mybook.to/empoweredADHDbook

resources

ADDitude Editors, & Panel, A. A. M. R. (2023, February 8). *Why Sugar is Kryptonite: ADHD Diet Truths.* ADDitude. https://www.additudemag.com/adhd-diet-nutrition-sugar/

ADHD and diet. (2022, September 22). Tees Esk and Wear Valley NHS Foundation Trust. https://www.tewv.nhs.uk/about-your-care/conditions/adhd/diet/

ADHD Diet and Nutrition. (2008, May 13). WebMD. https://www.webmd.com/add-adhd/adhd-diets

Amen, D. G. (2016). *Change Your Brain Change Your Life: The Breakthrough Programme for Conquering Anxiety, Depression, Anger and Obsessiveness.* Little, Brown Book Group Limited.

Barnes, Z., & Byrne, C. (2023, February 6). *7 Zinc Benefits Every Woman Should Know About. Women's Health.* https://www.womenshealthmag.com/food/g19967379/signs-youre-not-getting-zinc/

Chevallier, A. (2018). *Herbal Remedies Handbook: More Than 140 Plant Profiles; Remedies for Over 50 Common Conditions.* Dorling Kindersley Limited.

Engels, J. (2022, April 18). *Plant-Based Foods With the Highest Omega-3 Fatty Acids*. One Green Planet. https://www.onegreenplanet.org/natural-health/plant-based-foods-with-the-highest-amount-of-omega-3-fatty-acids/

Harvard Health. (2021, March 6). *Foods linked to better brainpower*. https://www.health.harvard.edu/healthbeat/foods-linked-to-better-brainpower

Harvard Health Publishing Staff. (2022, January 19). *How much protein do you need every day?* Harvard Health. https://www.health.harvard.edu/blog/how-much-protein-do-you-need-every-day-201506188096

Healthy Food Guide. (2021, September 22). *How much meat is healthy to eat?* https://www.healthyfood.com/advice/how-much-meat-is-healthy-to-eat/

Hjalmarsdottir, M. F. S. (2023, January 17). *17 Science-Based Benefits of Omega-3 Fatty Acids*. Healthline. https://www.healthline.com/nutrition/17-health-benefits-of-omega-3

Huizen, J. (2019, November 1). *All you need to know about egg yolk*. https://www.medicalnewstoday.com/articles/320445

Kubala, M. J. S. (2019, August 20). *7 Science-Based Health Benefits of Selenium*. Healthline. https://www.healthline.com/nutrition/selenium-benefits

Nelson, J. B. (2017, August 1). *Mindful Eating: The Art of Presence While You Eat*. American Diabetes Association. https://diabetesjournals.org/spectrum/article/30/3/171/32398/Mindful-Eating-The-Art-of-Presence-While-You-Eat

NHS website. (2022, September 13). *Eating processed foods*. nhs.uk. https://www.nhs.uk/live-well/eat-well/how-to-eat-a-balanced-diet/what-are-processed-foods/

Pelsser, L.M.J., Frankena, K., Toorman, J. *et al.* A randomised controlled trial into the effects of food on ADHD. *Eur Child Adolesc Psychiatry* 18, 12–19 (2009). https://doi.org/10.1007/s00787-008-0695-7

Shareghfarid, E., Sangsefidi, Z. S., Salehi-Abargouei, A., & Hosseinzadeh, M. (2020). Empirically derived dietary patterns and food groups intake in relation with Attention Deficit/Hyperactivity Disorder (ADHD): A systematic review and meta-analysis. *Clinical Nutrition ESPEN*, *36*, 28-35. https://doi.org/10.1016/j.clnesp.2019.10.013

Streit, M. L. S. (2020, December 2). *8 High Protein Nuts to Add to Your Diet*. Healthline. https://www.healthline.com/nutrition/high-protein-nuts

U. (2022, September 6). *The Surprising Health Benefits of Magnesium*. University Hospitals. https://www.uhhospitals.org/blog/articles/2022/09/the-surprising-health-benefits-of-magnesium

www.ingramcontent.com/pod-product-compliance
Lightning Source LLC
Chambersburg PA
CBHW060033040426
42333CB00042B/2407